The Everyda
101 Family-Fr
Inspired by The Mediterranean Diet

MW01233893

by **Vesela Tabakova**
Text copyright(c)2013 Vesela Tabakova
All Rights Reserved

Table Of Contents

What is the Paleo Diet and Does It Really Work?

The Paleo Diet is one of the best known diets nowadays, probably because it achieves great results. One can eat a variety of foods and it is good for the overall health – not only for losing weight. Whenever I want to lose a few pounds and fit into my jeans, I go strictly Paleo for a few weeks and I always see good results. The diet is all over the news, magazines and the web, so you probably know what it is all about – it mimics the types of foods people ate prior to the Agricultural Revolution about 10,000 years ago when they were still hunters and gatherers. That's why the foods you can eat on a paleo regime must be foods that you can gather or find, hunt or fish. Refined sugars and grains, dairy, and processed foods that often cause weight gain, diabetes and many other health problems are not allowed when you follow the paleolithic diet.

The main reason I'm a big fan of Paleo eating is because you can eat what you want (provided it is Paleo), and whenever you feel like eating. You don't stress over counting calories and you can eat as much as you want from the allowed foods – yet you still lose weight. The Paleo Diet works for me, because once I stop eating refined sugar, wheat, rice and other grains and starches, I always lose a few pounds. It also works because I have an enormous choice of vegetables and don't have to give up my favorite fruits. Following the Paleo Diet I don't feel deprived and always hungry, I eat lots of nuts and seeds as snacks and I can still prepare healthy meals for my family and eat them without feeling deprived and miserable.

These are my usual Paleo recipes when I choose to follow the Paleo Diet. I admit that I cannot follow this diet for an extended period of time but whenever I eat and cook for the Paleo Diet, I am very strict – I include only foods I am absolutely sure are allowed – no controversial grains, legumes or dairy products. I hope you will enjoy my recipes and together we will take a step towards healthier living.

Foods You Can Eat and Enjoy While on the Paleo Diet

One of the hardest things when you are on a diet is to avoid eating the same foods day after day. When you get bored with what you eat you are one step away from failing and returning to your old eating habits. So this list will give you some ideas as to what to prepare to please yourself and your family, and it will broaden your food choices.

The Paleo diet gives you the chance to try out some foods you don't normally choose and to experiment with meat and veggies or fruits that are less popular.

Meat - beef, veal, pork, sheep, lamb, rabbit, bison, wild boar, chicken, turkey, duck, quail, goose

Fish and shellfish– sardines, salmon, tuna, halibut, sole, trout, bass, haddock, turbot, tilapia, cod, mackerel, anchovy, herring, crab, lobster, shrimps, scallops, clams, oysters, mussels

Fats - avocado oil, olive oil, coconut oil, lard, duck fat, veal fat, lamb fat, nut butters, nut oils

Eggs -chicken eggs, duck eggs, goose eggs

Mushrooms - Button mushroom, oyster mushroom, portabello, shiitake, chanterelle, crimini, porcini

Vegetables - tomatoes, bell peppers, cucumbers, celery, onions, garlic, leeks, green onions, eggplants, cauliflower, broccoli, asparagus, cucumber, cabbage, Brussels sprouts, artichokes, okra, avocados, lettuce, spinach, collard greens, kale, beet greens, mustard greens, dandelion, Swiss chard, turnip greens, watercress, endive, rocket, radicchio, chicory, bok choy

Root vegetables -carrots, beetroot, turnip, parsnip, rutabaga, sweet potatoes, radishes, artichokes, yams, cassava

Winter and Summer Squash – pumpkin, butternut squash, zucchini, yellow summer squash

Fruit – apples, pears, peaches, nectarines, apricots, cherries, bananas, oranges, tangerine, grapefruit, strawberries, cranberries blueberries, blackberries, plums, pomegranates, pineapple, papaya, grapes, watermelon, honeydew melon, kiwis, lemon, lime, lychee, mango, coconut, figs, dates

Nuts and Seeds - sunflower seeds, pumpkin seeds, walnuts, pecans, pine nuts, macadamia nuts, chestnuts, cashews, almonds, sesame seeds, hazelnuts pistachios, Brazil nuts

Herbs - parsley, dill, oregano, rosemary, basil, thyme, bay leaves, lavender, mint, chives, tarragon, sage, coriander

Spices – paprika, savory, black pepper, fennel seeds, mustard seeds, cayenne pepper, cumin, turmeric, cinnamon, nutmeg, vanilla, cloves, ginger

Paleo Salads and Appetizers

Chicken and Egg Salad

Serves 6

Ingredients:

2 cups cooked chicken, chopped

2 hard boiled eggs, diced

2-3 pickled gherkins, chopped

1 large apple, diced

1/2 cup walnuts, baked

4 tbsp lemon juice

2 tbsp olive oil

salt and pepper, to taste

Directions:

Bake walnuts in a single layer in a preheated to 480 F oven for 3 minutes or until toasted and fragrant, stirring halfway through.

Stir together chicken, apple, eggs and gherkins. Combine lemon juice, olive oil, salt and pepper to taste and add to the chicken mixture. Sprinkle with walnuts and serve.

Chicken and Avocado Salad

Serves 4

Ingredients:

2 cups grilled skinless, boneless chicken breast, diced

2 avocados, peeled, pitted and diced

1 red onion, finely chopped

1/2 cup green olives, pitted

10 cherry tomatoes, halved

2 tbsp lemon juice

3 tbsp olive oil

1/2 tsp oregano

salt and black pepper, to taste

Directions:

In a medium bowl, combine the avocados, chicken, onion, and cherry tomatoes. Season with oregano, salt and pepper to taste.

Add the olives, lemon juice and olive oil and toss lightly to coat.

Greek Chicken Salad

Serves 4

Ingredients:

4 small chicken breast halves

Juice of one lemon

1-2 tsp fresh rosemary, chopped

3 garlic cloves, crushed

4 tbsp olive oil

2 tomatoes, cut into thin wedges

1 small red onion, cut into thin wedges

1/4 cup black olives, pitted

1/4 cup parsley leaves, chopped

Directions:

Prepare a dressing from the lemon juice, garlic, rosemary and olive oil. Place chicken fillets in a bowl with half the dressing. Stir well and marinate for at least 15 minutes.

Heat a char-grill pan or non-stick frying pan over medium high heat. Cook the chicken for five minutes each side until golden and cooked through. Set aside, covered with foil.

Toss the tomatoes, onion, olives and parsley in the remaining dressing. Slice the chicken thickly and add to the salad, then toss gently to combine.

Chicken and Lettuce Salad

Serves 6-7

Ingredients:

2 cups cooked chicken, coarsely chopped

1/2 head iceberg lettuce, sliced and chopped

1 celery rib, chopped

1 medium apple, cut

1/2 red bell pepper, deseeded and chopped

6-7 green olives, pitted and halved

1 red onion, chopped

for the dressing:

1 tbsp raw honey

2 tbsp lemon juice

salt and pepper, to taste

Directions:

Cut all the vegetables and toss them together with the olives in a large bowl.

Chop the already cooked and cooled chicken into small pieces and add it to the salad.

Prepare the salad dressing in a separate smaller bowl. Season with salt and pepper to taste and serve.

Italian Chicken Salad

Serves 4

Ingredients:

2 chicken breasts, cooked, shredded

2 yellow or orange bell peppers, thinly sliced

1 small red onion, thinly sliced

1 celery rib, chopped

1/4 cup slivered almonds, toasted

1 tbsp drained capers

juice of one lemon

1 tsp fresh thyme, minced

1/4 cup olive oil

salt and pepper, to taste

Directions:

Combine vegetables and chicken in a salad bowl.

Prepare a dressing by mixing the olive oil, lemon juice, thyme, salt and pepper, and pour over the salad.

Stir well to combine and serve.

Green Lettuce and Tuna Salad

Serves 4

Ingredients:

1 head green lettuce, washed and drained

1 cucumber, cut

1 can tuna, drained and broken into big chunks

a bunch of radishes, cut

a bunch of spring onions, finely cut

juice of half lemon or 2 tbsp of white wine vinegar

3 tbsp olive oil

salt to taste

Directions:

Cut the lettuce into thin strips. Slice the cucumber and the radishes as thinly as possible and chop the spring onions.

Mix all the vegetables in a large bowl, add the tuna and season with lemon juice, oil and salt to taste.

Beetroot and Carrot Salad with Salmon and Egg

Serves 4

Ingredients:

3 eggs, boiled and quartered

2 beets, peeled and coarsely grated

2 carrots, peeled and coarsely grated

5 oz smoked salmon portions, flaked

3-4 spring onions, chopped

1/4 cup fresh lemon juice

2 tbsp olive oil

salt and black pepper, to taste

Directions:

Boil eggs over high heat for three minutes. Drain, cool and peel. Shred carrots and beets and divide them among serving plates. Cut each egg in quarters and place on top of the vegetables. Top with the salmon flakes.

Prepare the dressing by whisking lemon juice and oil in a small bowl. Season with salt and pepper and drizzle over the salad. Serve sprinkled with spring onions.

Warm Italian Beef and Spinach Salad

Serves 4

Ingredients:

8 oz deli Italian roast beef, cut into 1/4 inch strips

1 red onion, sliced and separated into rings

2 tomatoes, sliced

1 red bell pepper, sliced

6 cups baby spinach or torn fresh spinach leaves

2 tbsp olive oil

2 garlic cloves, crushed

2 tbsp lemon juice

Directions:

Stir together all dressing ingredients in a deep bowl and set aside.

Warm olive oil in a large skillet and sauté beef and onions. Cook for 3-4 minutes, stirring occasionally, over medium heat, until beef is heated through.

Toss together beef, spinach, tomatoes, red pepper, garlic and lemon juice in a large salad bowl.

Mediterranean Steak Salad

Serves 4

Ingredients:

1 lb boneless beef sirloin steak, 1 inch thick

4 cups, romaine or rocket leaves, torn

1 red onion, sliced and separated into rings

1 cup cherry tomatoes, halved

1/2 cup green olives, pitted

1 tsp salt

1/2 tsp black pepper

for the dressing:

3 garlic cloves, crushed

5 tbsp olive oil

5 tbsp lemon juice

1 tsp lemon zest

1/2 tsp dried thyme

Directions:

Prepare the dressing by combining all ingredients in a bowl.

Heat a heavy skillet. Season steak with 1 teaspoon salt and 1/2 teaspoon black pepper. Cook it for 3-4 minutes on medium heat then turn and cook 3-4 minutes more. Transfer steak to a cutting board and leave it to cool. Slice it thinly.

Divide romaine lettuce among 4 plates. Top with sliced meat, red onion, tomatoes and olives. Drizzle with the dressing.

Mediterranean Beef Salad

Serves 6

Ingredients:

8 oz roast beef, thinly sliced

6 cups assorted greens, torn

2 carrots, grated

6-7 fresh mushrooms, thinly sliced

4 tbsp fresh basil leaves, torn

Ba 2 tbsp lemon juice

4 tbsp olive oil

1 tsp salt

Directions:

Prepare the dressing by mixing lemon juice, olive oil, crushed garlic, salt and basil leaves in a bowl.

Divide greens among four plates. Arrange beef with vegetables and mushrooms on top. Drizzle with dressing.

Moroccan Lamb Salad with Roasted Vegetables and Baby Spinach

Serves 4

Ingredients:

1 lb lamb fillets, trimmed

4 cups baby spinach

2 onions, cut into rings

2 small eggplants

2 zucchinis

2 red bell peppers

2 tbsp olive oil

1 tsp drained capers

2 tsp dry mint

for the dressing

juice of 2-3 lemons

5 tbsp olive oil

Directions:

Rub lamb fillets with mint and olive oil and refrigerate for at least 1 hour. Season with salt and pepper, place on the grill and cook to taste.

Cut onions into rings, eggplants, zucchinis and peppers into slices, then rub with olive oil, season with salt and pepper, and grill until cooked.

Place baby spinach and grilled vegetables in a large mixing bowl and stir; add capers and dressing and combine again.

Place salad into plates, top with sliced lamb and serve.

Warm Lamb Salad

Serves 4

Ingredients:

1 lb lamb back strap

1 small lettuce, chopped

1 cucumber, thinly sliced

1 red onion, sliced

1 yellow pepper, sliced

1/2 cup green olives, pitted

1 tsp fresh mint, chopped

for the dressing

2 tbsp orange juice

1 tbsp lemon juice

2 tbsp olive oil

2 garlic cloves, crushed

Directions:

Combine lettuce, cucumber, onion, pepper and fresh mint in a salad bowl.

Prepare the dressing by mixing all ingredients.

Preheat chargrill on high and cook lamb for 3-4 minutes each side, or until cooked to taste. Set aside, covered, for 5 minutes.

Slice and toss through salad with dressing.

Mushroom Salad

Serves 4

Ingredients:

1 lb fresh mushrooms, sliced

for the dressing

2 tbsp lemon juice

3 tbsp olive oil

2 garlic cloves, crushed

1 tsp dry thyme, crushed

1 tsp dry oregano, crushed

1/4 tbsp black pepper

Directions:

Prepare the dressing by combining all ingredients in a medium bowl very well.

Add the mushrooms, toss to coat with dressing, and serve

Paleo Greek Salad

Serves 6

Ingredients:

2 cucumbers, diced

2 tomatoes, sliced

1 green lettuce, cut

2 red bell peppers, cut

1/2 cup black olives, pitted

1 red onion, sliced

2 tbsp olive oil

2 tbsp lemon juice

salt and ground black pepper, to taste

Directions:

Dice the cucumbers and slice the tomatoes. Tear the lettuce or cut it in thin strips. De-seed and cut the peppers in strips.

Mix all vegetables in a salad bowl. Add the olives.

In a small cup mix the olive oil and the lemon juice with salt and pepper.

Pour over the salad and stir again.

Avocado Appetizer

Serves 6

Ingredients:

2 large, ripe avocados, peeled and seeded

1 tomato, very finely cut

2 spring onions, very finely cut

1 garlic clove, crushed

juice of 1/2 lime

1/4 tsp chili powder (optional)

1/4 tsp salt

fresh cilantro to garnish, finely chopped

Directions:

Mash all ingredients in a bowl with a fork and serve immediately.

Roasted Eggplant and Pepper Relish

Serves 4

Ingredients:

2 medium eggplants

2 red or green bell peppers

2 tomatoes

3 cloves garlic, crushed

fresh parsley, to serve

1-2 tbsp lemon juice

olive oil, as needed

salt, pepper

Directions:

Wash and dry the vegetables. Prick the skin of the eggplants. Bake the eggplants, tomatoes and peppers in a pre-heated oven at 430 F for about 30 minutes, until the skins are pretty burnt.

Take out of the oven and leave in a covered container for about 10 minutes. Peel the skins off and drain well the extra juices. De-seed the peppers.

Cut all the vegetables into small pieces. Add the garlic and mix well with a fork or in a food processor. Add the olive oil, lemon juice and salt to taste. Stir again.

Serve cold and sprinkled with parsley.

Apple, Celery and Walnut Salad

Serves 4

Ingredients:

4 apples, quartered, cores removed, thinly sliced

1 celery rib, thinly sliced

1/2 cup walnuts, chopped

2 tbsp raisins

1 large red onion, thinly sliced

3 tbsp lemon juice

2 tbsp coconut oil

Directions:

Mix lemon juice, coconut oil, salt and pepper in a small bowl. Whisk until well combined.

Combine apples, celery, walnuts, raisins and onion in a large bowl. Drizzle with the dressing and toss gently to combine.

Asian Coleslaw

Serves 4

Ingredients:

for the salad:

1/2 Chinese cabbage, shredded

1 green bell pepper, sliced into thin strips

1 carrot, cut into thin strips

4 green onions, chopped

for the dressing

3 tbsp lemon juice

1 tbsp raw honey

1 tbsp olive oil

Directions:

Remove any damaged outer leaves and rinse cabbage. Holding cabbage from the base and starting at the opposite end shred leaves thinly.

Combine vegetables first then dressing ingredients. Pour over salad and toss well.

Asparagus Salad

Serves 4

Ingredients:

1 lb asparagus, ends trimmed, cut into 2 inch lengths

3-4 spring onions, chopped

2 tbsp olive oil

2 tbsp lemon juice

2 garlic cloves, chopped

salt, to taste

black pepper, to taste

Directions:

Cook asparagus in boiling salted water for one to two minutes, or until bright green and tender. Drain and rinse.

Mix with all other ingredients. Combine olive oil, lemon juice, salt and black pepper and drizzle over the salad.

Serve chilled or at room temperature.

Baby Spinach Salad

Serves 4

Ingredients:

1 bag baby spinach, washed and dried

1 red bell pepper, cut in slices

1 cup cherry tomatoes, cut in halves

1 red onion, finely chopped

1 cup black olives, pitted

1 tsp dried oregano

1 large garlic clove, cut

3 tbsp lemon juice

4 tbsp olive oil

salt and freshly ground black pepper, to taste

Directions:

Prepare the dressing by blending the garlic and the oregano with the olive oil and the lemon juice in a food processor.

Place the spinach leaves in a large salad bowl and toss with the dressing. Add the rest of the ingredients and give everything a toss again.

Season to taste with black pepper and salt.

Fresh Greens Salad

Serves 8

Ingredients:

1 head red leaf lettuce, rinsed, dried and chopped

1 head green leaf lettuce, rinsed, dried, and chopped

1 head endive, rinsed, dried and chopped

1 cup frisee lettuce leaves, rinsed, dried, and chopped

3 leaves fresh basil, chopped

3 sprigs fresh mint, chopped

4 tbsp olive oil

2 tbsp lemon juice

salt, to taste

Directions:

Place the red and green leaf lettuce, frisee lettuce, endive, basil and mint into a large salad bowl and toss lightly to combine.

Prepare the dressing from lemon juice and olive oil and pour over the salad.

Season with salt to taste.

Paleo Fatoush

Serves 6

Ingredients:

2 cups green lettuce, washed, dried, and chopped

3 tomatoes, chopped

1 cucumber, peeled and chopped

1 green pepper, seeded and chopped

1/2 cup radishes, sliced in half

1 small red onion, finely chopped

half a bunch of parsley, finely cut

2 tbsp finely chopped fresh mint

3 tbsp olive oil

4 tbsp lemon juice

salt and black pepper, to taste

Directions:

Place the lettuce, tomatoes, cucumbers, green pepper, radishes, onion, parsley and mint in a salad bowl.

Make the dressing by whisking together the olive oil with the lemon juice, a pinch of salt, and some black pepper.

Toss everything together until everything is coated with dressing and serve.

Green Lettuce Salad

Serves 4

Ingredients:

, 1 green lettuce, washed and drained

1 cucumber

a bunch of radishes

a bunch of spring onions

the juice of half a lemon

3 tbsp coconut or olive oil

salt to taste

Directions:

Cut the lettuce into thin strips. Slice the cucumber and the radishes as thinly as possible and chop the spring onions.

Mix all the salad ingredients in a large bowl, add the lemon juice and oil and season with salt to taste.

Red Cabbage Salad

Serves 6

Ingredients:

1 small head red cabbage, cored and chopped

a bunch of fresh dill, finely cut

3 tbsp coconut oil

3 tbsp lemon juice

2 tbsp salt

black pepper, to taste

Directions:

In a bowl, mix the oil, lemon juice and black pepper. Place the cabbage in a large salad bowl. Sprinkle the salt on top and crunch it with your hands to soften.

Pour dressing over the cabbage and toss to coat. Sprinkle the salad with dill, cover it with foil and leave it in the refrigerator for half an hour before serving.

Okra Salad

Serves 4

Ingredients:

1 lb young okras

1 lemon

1/2 bunch of parsley, chopped

2 hard tomatoes, cut into slices

3 tbsp coconut oil

1/2 tsp black pepper

salt, to taste

Directions:

Trim okras, wash and cook in salted water. Drain and cool when tender.

In a small bowl mix well the lemon juice and coconut oil, salt and pepper. Pour over okras arranged in a bowl and sprinkle with chopped parsley.

Wash tomatoes and cut them into slices, then garnish the salad with them.

Cucumber Salad

Serves 4

Ingredients:

2 medium cucumbers, sliced

a bunch of fresh dill

2 cloves garlic

3 tbsp lemon juice

3 tbsp olive oil

salt to taste

Directions:

Cut the cucumbers in rings and arrange them in a plate.

Add the finely cut dill, the pressed garlic and season with salt, vinegar and oil. Mix well and serve cold.

Beetroot Salad

Serves 4

Ingredients:

2-3 small beets, peeled

3 spring onions, chopped

3 garlic cloves, pressed

2 tbsp lemon juice

2-3 tbsp coconut oil

salt to taste

Directions:

Place the beats in a steam basket set over a pot of boiling water. Steam them for about 15-20 minutes, or until tender. Leave to cool.

Grate the beets and put them in a salad bowl. Add the crushed garlic cloves, the finely cut spring onions and toss to combine.

Season with salt, vinegar and coconut oil.

Carrot Salad

Serves 4

Ingredients:

4 carrots, shredded

1 apple, peeled, cored and shredded

2 garlic cloves, crushed

2 tbsp lemon juice

salt and pepper, to taste

Directions:

In a bowl, combine the shredded carrots, apple, lemon juice, garlic, salt and pepper.

Toss and chill before serving.

Eggplant and Pepper Salad

Serves 4

Ingredients:

2 medium eggplants

2 red or green bell peppers

4-5 cloves garlic, crushed

a bunch of fresh parsley

1-2 tbsp lemon juice

4 tbsp olive oil

salt, pepper

Directions:

Grill the peppers and the eggplants or roast them in the oven at 480 F until the skins are a little burnt. Place them in a brown paper bag or a lidded container and leave covered for about 10 minutes. This makes it easier to peel the skins. Peel them and remove the seeds.

Cut the peppers and the eggplants into 1 inch strips lengthwise and layer them in a bowl.

Mix together the oil, lemon juice, salt and pepper, chopped garlic and the chopped parsley leaves. Pour over the vegetables.

Cover the roasted peppers and eggplants and chill for an hour. Serve.

Paleo Soup Recipes

Paleo Chicken Soup

Serves 8

Ingredients:

about 1 lb chicken breasts

3-4 carrots, chopped

1 celery rib, chopped

1 red onion, chopped

8 cups water

10 black olives, pitted and halved

fresh parsley or coriander, to serve

1/2 tsp salt

ground black pepper, to taste

lemon juice, to serve

Directions:

Place chicken breasts in a soup pot. Add onion, carrots, celery, salt, pepper and water. Stir well and bring to a boil. Add olives, stir and reduce heat. Simmer for 30-40 minutes.

Remove chicken from pot and let it cool slightly. Shred it and return it to pot.

Serve soup with lemon juice and sprinkled with fresh parsley or coriander.

Moroccan Chicken and Butternut Squash Soup

Serves 8

Ingredients:

3 skinless, boneless chicken thighs (about 14 oz), cut into bite-sized pieces

1 big onion, chopped

1 zucchini, quartered lengthwise and sliced into 1/2-inch pieces

3 cups peeled butternut squash, cut in 1/2-inch pieces

2 tbsp tomato paste

4 cups chicken broth

1/2 tsp ground cumin

1/4 tsp ground cinnamon

1 tsp paprika

1 tsp salt

2 tbsp fresh basil leaves, chopped

1 tbsp grated orange rind

3 tbsp olive oil

Directions:

Heat a soup pot over medium heat. Gently sauté onion, for 3-4 minutes, stirring occasionally. Add chicken pieces and cook for 4 minutes, until chicken is brown on all sides.

Add cumin, cinnamon and paprika and stir well. Add butternut squash and tomato paste; stir again. Add chicken broth and bring to a boil then reduce heat, and simmer 10 minutes.

Stir in salt and zucchini pieces; cook until squash is tender.

Remove pot from heat. Season with salt and pepper to taste. Stir in chopped basil and orange rind and serve.

Balkan Chicken Soup

Serves 6-7

Ingredients:

1 whole chicken (3-4 lbs), cut into sections

1 large onion, whole

1 large onion, chopped

3 garlic cloves, chopped

2 carrots, chopped

1 red bell pepper

1 tsp thyme

2 bay leaves

2 tbsp olive oil

1 tsp salt

black pepper to taste

1 tsp savory

Directions:

Place the chicken, bay leaves, salt, whole onion and whole red pepper into a pot with five cups of cold water. Bring the pot to boil, reduce heat and simmer for one hour, scooping out any solid foam that settles at the top. When ready, strain the broth and reserve.

Remove the meat from the chicken and cut into large chunks. Discard the bay leaves, the onion and the pepper. Place the pot back on the stove, heat the olive oil and sauté the other onion, garlic, carrots and thyme for about 5 minutes.

Pour in the broth and season with salt and pepper. Simmer for about 15 minutes or until the vegetables are tender.

Add in the chicken pieces and the oregano. Simmer for 10 more minutes and serve warm.

Beef and Vegetable Soup

Serves 5-6

Ingredients:

2 lbs stewing beef

3 tbsp olive oil

1 large onion, chopped

1 cup mushrooms, chopped

2 carrots, chopped

1 celery rib, chopped

6 cups water

2 tbsp tomato paste

1/2 cup parsley, chopped

salt and black pepper, to taste

Directions:

Season the beef pieces with salt and pepper. In a large soup pot, heat olive oil and seal the beef in batches then set it aside in a plate, covered. Sauté the onions, mushrooms, carrots, and celery over medium high heat.

Return the meat to the pot, add water and bring to the boil. Reduce heat and simmer, covered, for about an hour, stirring occasionally.

Dissolve the tomato paste in a few tablespoons of the soup broth and add it to the pot. Stir in the chopped parsley and season with salt and pepper to taste.

Paleo Beef and Vegetable Minestrone

Serves 4-5

Ingredients:

2 slices bacon, chopped

1 cup ground beef

2 carrots, chopped

2 cloves garlic, finely chopped

1 large onion, chopped

1 celery rib, chopped

1 bay leaf

1 tsp dried basil

1 tsp dried rosemary, crushed

1/4 tsp crushed chillies

1 can tomatoes, chopped

4 cups beef broth

Directions:

In a large saucepan, cook bacon and ground beef until well done, breaking up the beef as it cooks. Drain off the fat and add carrots, garlic, onion and celery.

Cook for about 5 minutes or until the onions are translucent. Season with the bay leaf, basil, rosemary and crushed chillies. Stir in the tomatoes and beef broth.

Bring to a boil then reduce heat and simmer for about 30 minutes.

Italian Meatball Soup

Serves 8

Ingredients:

1 lb lean ground beef

1 small onion, grated

1 onion, chopped

2 garlic cloves, crushed

1 zucchini, diced

3-4 basil leaves, finely chopped

1 egg, lightly beaten

2 cups tomato sauce with basil

3 cups water

2 tbsp olive oil

salt and black pepper, to taste

Directions:

Combine ground meat, grated onion, garlic, basil and egg in a large bowl. Season with salt and pepper. Mix well with hands and roll tablespoonfuls of the mixture into balls. Place on a large plate.

Heat olive oil into a large deep saucepan and sauté onion and garlic until transparent. Add tomato sauce, water and bring to the boil over high heat. Add meatballs.

Reduce heat to medium-low and simmer, uncovered, for 10 minutes.

Paleo Meatball Soup

Serves 4-5

Ingredients:

1 lb lean ground beef

1 onion, chopped

2 garlic cloves, cut

1 tomato, diced

1 carrot, diced

1 green pepper, chopped

4 cups water

½ bunch of parsley, finely cut

3 tbsp olive oil

½ tsp black pepper

1 tsp savory

1 tsp paprika

1 tsp salt

Directions:

Combine ground meat, savory, paprika, black pepper and salt in a large bowl. Mix well with hands and roll teaspoonfuls of the mixture into balls.

Heat olive oil into a large soup pot and sauté onion and garlic until transparent. Add water and bring to the boil over high heat. Add the meatballs, carrot and green pepper. R

educe heat to low and simmer, uncovered, for 15 minutes. Add the tomato and the parsley and cook for 5 more minutes. Serve with lemon juice.

Spanish Seafood Soup

Serves 10

Ingredients:

2 lbs whole raw prawns

1 lb mussels

4 cups cold water

3 spring onions, chopped

1 bell pepper, finely chopped

2 large tomatoes, diced

1 tbsp tomato puree

2 garlic cloves, minced

2 tbsp olive oil

2 bay leaves

1 tsp paprika

½ tsp cayenne pepper

salt and pepper to taste

the juice of one small lemon

a bunch of parsley, chopped

Directions:

De-head and de-shell the prawns and leave them in a bowl to the side. Put the heads and shells in a pan with cold water. Add the bay leaves, bring to the boil and reduce heat.

Simmer for 20 minutes. While the broth is simmering, sauté the shallots and pepper in olive oil for 5 minutes, then add the garlic for two more minutes.

When the broth is ready strain it and add it to the the shallots. Bring to the boil, add the tomatoes and tomato puree, the prawns, the mussels and simmer for 10 more minutes.

In the end add the paprika and cayenne pepper, season to taste with salt and pepper and add the lemon juice.

Garnish with parsley and serve.

Hot Spanish Squid Soup

Serves 4

Ingredients:

1 lb Squid; cleaned, cut into 1 inch pieces

2 garlic cloves; crushed

1/2 cup tomato puree or chopped tomatoes

3 cups water

1 tbsp olive oil

black pepper, to taste

1/2 cup parsley, finely chopped, to serve

Directions:

Heat olive oil in a soup pot over medium high heat and gently sauté garlic just for a minute.

Add squid and sauté for 2-3 minutes, stirring. Add black pepper, tomato sauce or tomatoes and water.

Bring to a boil and let simmer soup for an hour. Serve sprinkled with parsley.

Lamb Soup

Serves 8

Ingredients:

2 lb lean boneless lamb, cubed

1 onion, finely cut

1 carrot, chopped

10 spring onions, chopped

2 tomato, diced

4 cups hot water

2 tbsp olive oil

1/2 tsp paprika

1 tsp salt

black pepper, to taste

1 tbsp dry mint

1/2 cup parsley, finely cut

2 eggs

Directions:

Heat olive oil and gently brown the lamb cubes in a medium sized cooking pot. Add the finely cut onion and the carrot and sauté for a minute or two, stirring. Add paprika and two cups of hot water.

Bring to the boil, then lower heat to medium-low and simmer until the lamb softens. Add in 2 more cups of hot water, spring onions, tomato, mint, salt and black pepper.

Bring to a boil again and simmer for 10 minutes.

53

Whisk the the eggs in a small bowl. Take one ladle from the soup and add into the egg mixture, whisk. Take another and whisk again.

Pour this mixture back into into the soup and stir. Do not boil. Sprinkle with parsley and serve while still hot.

Pumpkin and Bell Pepper Soup

Serves 4

Ingredients:

1 medium leek, chopped

9 oz pumpkin, peeled, deseeded, cut into small cubes

1/2 red bell pepper, cut into small pieces

1 can tomatoes, undrained, crushed

3 cups vegetable broth

1/2 tsp ground cumin

salt and black pepper, to taste

Directions:

Heat the olive oil in a medium saucepan and sauté the leek for 4-5 minutes. Add the pumpkin and bell pepper and cook, stirring, for 2-3 minutes. Add tomatoes, broth and cumin and bring to the boil.

Cover, reduce heat to low and simmer, stirring occasionally, for 30 minutes or until vegetables are soft.

Season with salt and pepper and leave aside to cool. Blend in batches and re-heat to serve.

Spicy Carrot Soup

Serves 6-7

Ingredients:

10 carrots, peeled and chopped

2 medium onions, chopped

4-5 cups water

5 tbsp coconut oil

2 cloves garlic, minced

1 red chili pepper, finely chopped

1/2 bunch, fresh coriander, finely cut

salt and pepper, to taste

Directions:

Heat the coconut oil in a large pot over medium heat, and sauté the onions, carrots, garlic and chili pepper until tender. Add 4-5 cups of water and bring to a boil. Reduce heat to low, and simmer 30 minutes.

Transfer the soup to a blender or food processor and blend until smooth. Return to the pot, and continue cooking for a few more minutes.

Remove soup from heat, and set aside for a few minutes. Serve with coriander sprinkled over each serving.

Mushroom Soup

Serves 4

Ingredients:

2 cups mushrooms, peeled and chopped

1 onion, chopped

2 cloves of garlic, crushed and chopped

1 tsp dried thyme

3 cups vegetable broth

salt and pepper to taste

3 tbsp coconut or olive oil

Directions:

Sauté onions and garlic in a large soup pot until transparent. Add thyme and mushrooms.

Cook, stirring, for 10 minutes then add vegetable broth and simmer for another 10-20 minutes. Blend, season and serve.

Tomato Soup

Serves: 5-6

Ingredients:

4 cups chopped fresh tomatoes or 2 cups canned tomatoes

1 large onion, diced

4 garlic cloves, minced

3 tbsp olive or coconut oil

2 cups hot water

1 tsp paprika

1 tsp dried basil

1 tsp salt

1/2 tsp black pepper

1 tsp raw honey

1/2 bunch fresh parsley

Directions:

Sauté the onions and garlic in oil in a large soup pot. When the onions have softened, add paprika and tomatoes and cook until onions are golden and tomatoes soft.

Stir in the spices and mix well to coat vegetables. Add one cup of hot water. Blend the soup then return to the pot. Add a tsp of raw honey and bring to boil, then simmer 20-30 minutes stirring occasionally.

Sprinkle with parsley and serve.

Creamless Cauliflower Soup

Serves 4-5

Ingredients:

1 large onion finely cut

1 medium head cauliflower, chopped

2-3 garlic cloves, minced

4 cups water

4 tbsp olive oil

salt, to taste

fresh ground black pepper, to taste

Directions:

Heat the olive oil in a large pot over medium heat, and sauté the onion, cauliflower, garlic, Stir in the water, and bring the soup to a boil.

Reduce heat, cover, and simmer for 40 minutes. Remove the soup from heat and blend in a blender.

Season with salt and black pepper to taste.

Roasted Red Pepper Soup

Serves 6-7

Ingredients:

5-6 red peppers

1 large onion, chopped

2 garlic cloves, crushed

4 medium tomatoes, chopped

4 cups vegetable broth

3 tbsp olive oil

2 bay leaves

Directions:

Grill the peppers or roast them in the oven at 480 F until the skins are a little burnt. Place the roasted peppers in a brown paper bag or a lidded container and leave covered for about 10 minutes. This makes it easier to peel them. Peel the skins and remove the seeds. Cut the peppers in small pieces.

Heat oil in a large saucepan over medium-high heat. Add onion and garlic and sauté, stirring, for 3 minutes or until onion has softened. Add the red peppers, bay leaves, tomato and simmer for 5 minutes.

Add broth. Season with pepper. Bring to the boil then reduce heat and simmer for 20 minutes. Set aside to cool slightly. Blend, in batches, until smooth and serve.

Lemon Artichoke Soup

Serves 6

Ingredients:

2 cups artichoke hearts, chopped

1 small onion, very finely cut

1 celery rib, very finely cut

2 carrots, very finely cut

1 garlic clove, crushed

3 cups chicken broth

2 tbsp olive oil

1 tsp salt

1 tsp black pepper

1 fresh lemon, halved

2 cups coconut milk

Directions:

Heat olive oil in a large pot and gently sauté onion, celery, carrot and garlic. Stir in chicken broth, artichokes, salt and pepper and bring to the boil. Lower heat and simmer for 10 minutes.

Remove from heat and blend until smooth. Return to heat, juice half a lemon into soup. Bring to the boil, reduce heat and simmer for 5 more minutes.

Stir in coconut milk and simmer for another 5 minutes.

Spinach Soup

Serves 6

Ingredients:

1 lb spinach, frozen

1 large onion or 4-5 spring onions

1 carrot

1 tomato, chopped

3 cups water

3-4 tbsp olive oil

1-2 cloves garlic, crushed

1 tsp paprika

black pepper

salt, to taste

Directions:

Chop the onion and the spinach. Heat the olive oil in a cooking pot, add the onion and carrot and sauté together for a few minutes, until just softened. Add chopped garlic and paprika and stir for a minute.

Remove from heat. Add the spinach, the tomato and about 2 cups of hot water and season with salt and pepper.

Bring back to the boil, then reduce the heat and simmer for about 15 minutes.

Paleo Nettle Soup

Serves 6

Ingredients:

1.5 lb young top shoots of nettles, well washed

1 cup spinach leaves

1 carrot, chopped

a bunch of spring onions, coarsely chopped

3 tbsp coconut oil

3 cups hot water

1 tsp salt

Directions:

Clean the young nettles, wash and cook them in slightly salted water. Drain, rinse, drain again and then chop or pass through a sieve.

Sauté the chopped spring onions and carrot in the oil until the onion softens. Add the nettles, the spinach leaves and gradually stir in the water.

Bring to a boil, reduce heat and simmer for 5 minutes. Set aside to cool then blend in batches.

Gazpacho

Serves 6-7

Ingredients:

6-7 medium tomatoes, peeled and halved

1 onion, sliced

1 green pepper, sliced

1 big cucumber, peeled and sliced

2 cloves garlic

salt to taste

4 tbsp olive oil

to garnish

1/2 onion, chopped

1 green pepper, chopped

1 cucumber, chopped

Directions:

Place the tomatoes, garlic, onion, green pepper, cucumber, salt and olive oil in a blender or food processor and puree until smooth, adding small amounts of cold water if needed to achieve desired consistency.

Serve the gazpacho chilled with the chopped onion, green pepper and cucumber.

Avocado Gazpacho

Serves 4

Ingredients:

2 ripe avocados, peeled, pitted and diced

1 cup tomatoes, diced

1 cup cucumbers, peeled and diced

1 small onion, chopped

2 tbsp lemon juice

1 tsp salt

black pepper, to taste

Directions:

Place avocados, cucumbers, tomatoes, onion, lemon juice and salt and pepper in a blender.

Blend until smooth and serve sprinkled with cilantro or parsley leaves.

Paleo Main and Side Dishes

Paleo Chicken and Vegetables

Serves 4

Ingredients:

4 skinless, boneless chicken breast halves

10 big mushrooms, whole

1 onion, sliced

2 carrots, cut

1 red bell pepper, halved, deseeded, cut

1 zucchini, cut

4 garlic cloves, thinly sliced

1 cup water

3 tbsp olive oil

1 tsp dry oregano

Directions:

Preheat oven to 350 F. Heat oil in a non stick frying pan over medium heat. Cook half the chicken, turning occasionally, for 5 minutes or until brown all over. Set aside. Repeat with the remaining chicken.

Peel and cut the carrots and the zucchini. Cut the onion and the pepper. Transfer chicken to a roasting pan. Add vegetables and mushrooms on and around the chicken. Add dried oregano, garlic and water, distributing evenly across the pan.

Roast uncovered at 350 F for one hour. Half way through stir gently. If needed, add a little more water.

Chicken and Onion Stew

Serves 4

Ingredients:

4 chicken breast halves

4-5 big onions, thinly sliced

1/2 cup black olives, pitted

4 tbsp olive oil

1 tsp thyme

1 tsp turmeric

salt and black pepper to taste

1/4 cup parsley leaves, chopped, to serve

Directions:

Heat the oil in a large, deep, frying pan over medium-high heat. Cook chicken, turning, for 4 to 5 minutes or until golden. Transfer to a plate.

Sauté thinly sliced onions, stirring gently, for 5 minutes until soft. Add olives, thyme, turmeric, salt and pepper to taste. Return chicken to the pan.

Cover and bring to the boil. Reduce heat to low and simmer for 35 minutes or until chicken is cooked through. Sprinkle with parsley and serve.

Chicken and Mushroom Stew

Serves 4

Ingredients:

4 chicken breast halves, cut into bite size pieces

1 lb mushrooms, sliced (5-6 cups)

1 bunch of spring onions, chopped

4 tbsp olive oil

1 tsp thyme

salt and black pepper to taste

Directions:

Heat oil in a large, deep, frying pan over medium high heat. Cook chicken, stirring, for 4-5 minutes or until golden. Add spring onions, mushrooms, salt and pepper and stir.

Cover and bring to the boil. Reduce heat to low and simmer for 25 minutes.

Paleo Chicken Casserole

Serves 4

Ingredients:

4 skinless, boneless chicken breast halves or 8 tights

1 lb okra

1 big onion, chopped

2 cups diced, canned tomatoes, undrained

5 garlic cloves, crushed

1 tsp paprika

salt and black pepper to taste

Directions:

Preheat oven to 350 F. Heat oil in a large baking dish over medium heat. Add onion and sauté for 2 minutes. Add paprika, black pepper and garlic and sauté for another minute. Stir in okra and tomatoes.

Remove from heat. Arrange chicken pieces into the vegetables, sprinkle with salt and pepper.

Cover and bake for 40 minutes, stirring gently halfway through.

Chicken and Zucchini Moussaka

Serves: 4

Ingredients:

2-3 zucchinis, peeled and cut into thick rounds

1 tbsp salt

1 onion, finely cut

2 garlic cloves, crushed

1/2 tsp ground nutmeg

1/4 tsp ground coriander

1/4 tsp ground ginger

1 can tomatoes, undrained, chopped

2 cups cooked chicken, shredded

1 cup parsley leaves, finely chopped

2 eggs

3 tbsp coconut milk

4 tbsp olive oil

salt and black pepper, to taste

Directions:

Peel and slices the zucchinis. Sprinkle them with a tablespoon of salt and set aside for 30 minutes. Rinse and pat dry.

In a deep frying, heat olive oil over medium-high heat and fry the zucchinis for 2-3 minutes each side or until golden. Set aside in a plate.

In the same pan, gently sauté onion and garlic until fragrant. Add in all spices and sauté for 1-2 minutes more. Add in tomatoes and simmer until the tomato sauce thickness. Add chicken, parsley and stir to combine.

Arrange half the zucchinis in an ovenproof baking dish. Cover with chicken and tomato mixture and top with remaining zucchinis.

Whisk two eggs with coconut milk. Pour over the meat and zucchini mixture.

Bake for 35 minutes or until golden. Set aside for five minutes and serve.

Hunter Style Chicken

Serves 4-6

Ingredients:

1 chicken (3-4 lbs), cut into pieces

2 tbsp olive or coconut oil

3 medium onions, thinly sliced

2 red bell peppers, cut

6-7 white mushrooms, sliced

2 cups canned tomatoes, diced and drained

3 garlic cloves, thinly sliced

salt and freshly ground pepper

1/2 cup parsley leaves, finely cut

Directions:

Rinse chicken pieces and pat dry. Heat olive oil in a large skillet on medium heat. Working in batches cook the chicken pieces until nicely browned, 5-6 minutes, then turn over and brown the other side.

Transfer chicken to a bowl, set aside. Drain off all of the rendered fat.

Add 2 tbsp of olive oil and sauté the sliced onions and bell peppers for a few minutes. Add the mushrooms and cook some more until onion is translucent. Add garlic and tomatoes and cook a minute more.

Place the chicken pieces on top of the vegetables, skin side up. Lower the heat and cover the skillet with the lid slightly ajar.

time, until the meat is almost falling off the bones. Sprinkle with parsley, set aside for 3-4 minutes and serve.

Small Chicken Meatballs

Serves 4

Ingredients:

1 lb ground chicken meat

1 onion, grated

2 medium tomatoes, diced

1 egg, lightly whisked

3 tbsp chopped parsley leaves

1 tbs freshly ground ginger

1/2 tsp ground cinnamon

1/2 tsp ground nutmeg

2 tbsp olive oil

1/2 cup chicken broth

1 tbsp lemon juice

Directions:

Preheat the oven to 350 F. Line a baking tray with baking paper.

Place the ground chicken, onion, egg, chopped parsley, cinnamon, nutmeg and half the ginger in a bowl with a teaspoon of salt. Mix with your hands until well combined.

Using damp hands, roll mixture into walnut-sized balls, then place them on a tray in a single layer and bake for 15 minutes until light golden.

Heat oil in a deep frying pan over medium heat. Add remaining ginger and stir for 1 minute until fragrant. Add tomatoes and cook for 2 minutes. Add broth.

Bring to a boil, then reduce heat to medium low and simmer for 5 minutes. Add meatballs and simmer for 20 minutes until they are cooked through and the sauce has thickened.

Serve garnished with extra parsley.

Grilled Chicken with Sumac

Serves 4

Ingredients:

1 whole chicken(3-4 lbs)

2 tbsp olive oil

2 garlic cloves, crushed

1 tbsp sumac

1 tsp lemon zest

1 tbsp lemon juice

1/2 cup fresh coriander leaves

Directions:

Wash throughly chicken and pat dry with a paper towel.

Combine oil, garlic, sumac, lemon rind and lemon juice in a bowl. Rub mixture over chicken. Cover and marinate for 2 hours if time permits. Bake chicken in an oven proof dish, covered, for 1 hour.

Uncover and bake for 20 minutes more or until cooked through.

Cut chicken into large pieces and serve sprinkled with coriander and garnished with vegetable salads.

Chicken Skewers

Serves 4

Ingredients:

1.5 lb chicken breast fillets, cut in bite size pieces

3-4 tbsp coconut oil

2 garlic cloves, crushed

1 tsp paprika

1 tsp dried savory

Directions:

Thread chicken pieces onto skewers. Place in a shallow dish. Combine coconut oil and lemon juice, garlic, paprika and savory. Pour over chicken. Turn to coat. Marinate for 40 minutes, if time permits.

Preheat barbecue on medium high heat. Cook skewers for 3-4 minutes each side or until chicken is just cooked through. Serve with vegetable salad.

Moroccan Chicken Tagine

Serves 4-5

Ingredients:

1 whole chicken (3-4 lbs), cut into pieces

2 large onions, grated

2 or 3 cloves of garlic, finely chopped or pressed

1 tsp ginger

1 tsp cumin

1 tsp paprika

1 tsp black pepper

1 tsp turmeric

1/2 tsp salt

1/2 cup green or black olives, or mixed

1 preserved lemon, quartered and deseeded

5 tbsp olive oil

one bunch of fresh coriander

one bunch of fresh parsley

Directions:

Rinse and dry chicken and place onto a clean plate.

In a large bowl, mix three tablespoons of olive oil, salt, half the onions, garlic, ginger, cumin, paprika, and turmeric.

Mix thoroughly, crush the garlic with your fingers, and add a little water to make a paste.

Roll the chicken pieces into the marinade and leave for 10-15 minutes.

Heat the tagine base on medium heat and add 2 tablespoons of olive oil. Add the chicken and pour excess marinade juices over the top. Add the remaining onions, olives, and chopped preserved lemon. Tie the parsley and coriander together into a bouquet and place on top of the chicken.

Place the lid on the base, bring to a boil and immediately reduce to a simmer.

Cook for 45 minutes, or until the chicken is cooked through and quite tender.

Chicken Stir-Fry Omelette

Serves 4

Ingredients:

1/2 cup cooked chicken, shredded

3 eggs, beaten

1 carrot, chopped

2 garlic cloves, chopped

4 spring onions, chopped

1/2 cup Brussels sprouts, halved

1 tbsp olive oil

salt, to taste

Directions:

Heat olive oil in a large skillet over medium heat. Add carrot and garlic and stir fry for 1 minute.

Add Brussels sprouts and stir fry until soft. Add chicken, stir fry until heated through.

Add spring onions and eggs, salt to taste and scramble.

Spicy Mustard Chicken

Serves 4

Ingredients:

4 chicken breasts or 5-6 chicken tights

1/2 cup chicken broth

3-4 tbsp mustard

3 tbsp olive oil

1 tsp paprika

1 tsp chili powder

1 tsp garlic powder

Directions:

In a small bowl, mix mustard, olive oil, paprika, garlic powder, chicken broth, and chili. Marinate the chicken breasts for 30 minutes.

Bake on a lined baking sheet at 375 F for 35 minutes, turning once.

Lemon Chicken

Serves: 4

Ingredients:

4 chicken breasts

1 garlic clove, crushed

4 lemon slices

4-5 kalamata olives, pitted

1 tsp capers

1 tbsp dried rosemary

2 tbsp olive oil

1/2 tsp sumac

salt and pepper, to taste

Directions:

Heat the olive oil in a skillet over medium-low heat and gently sauté the garlic a minute, or until just fragrant.

Add in the lemon slices and lay the chicken breasts on top. Add capers, rosemary and olives.

Season with salt and pepper, cover the pan, and cook for 20 minutes or until the chicken breasts are cooked through, turning once.

Uncover and cook for 2-3 minutes, until all liquid evaporates.

Marinated Beef Skewers

Serves 4

Ingredients:

2 lbs beef, cut into 1 inch cubes

1 onion, chopped

4 garlic cloves, chopped

2 tbsp parsley, chopped

1 tbsp paprika

1/4 cup olive oil

1/4 cup orange juice

2 cups small mushrooms, whole

for the dressing:

2 tbsp lemon juice

1/4 cup olive oil

1 tbsp fresh rosemary leaves

Directions:

Place the beef cubes in a bowl together with the chopped onion and garlic. Add orange juice, paprika, parsley and olive oil. Mix thoroughly and marinate for at least an hour.

Thread beef onto skewers, dividing the cubes with mushrooms. Grill on a hot barbecue, turning, until cooked through.

Prepare the dressing by combining the lemon juice, olive oil and rosemary leaves.

Place skewers on plates and drizzle dressing on top. Serve with fresh salad.

Mediterranean Steak

Serves 4

Ingredients:

4 sirloin steaks, trimmed

6 large tomatoes, sliced

2 tsp baby capers

1/4 cup basil leaves

6 garlic cloves, whole

1 tbsp lemon juice

3 tbsp olive oil

salt and black pepper, to taste

olive oil spray

Directions:

Marinate the steaks in a glass bowl with half the olive oil, a tbsp lemon juice, salt and black pepper for 5 minutes.

Preheat oven to 350 F. Arrange tomatoes on a baking tray lined with baking paper. Scatter over capers and garlic cloves. Sprinkle with the remaining olive oil. Cook for 15 minutes. Remove and set aside.

Heat a grill pan over high heat. Cook the steaks for four minutes each side or until cooked through to you taste.

Serve steaks with roasted tomatoes and sprinkled with basil leaves.

Italian Roast Beef

Serves 6

Ingredients:

5 lb roast beef round

6 garlic cloves, sliced

4 onions, sliced

6 carrots, cut into rounds

4 celery ribs, cut into thick pieces

2 bay leaves

1 tbsp finely chopped rosemary

1/4 cup tomato paste

1/4 tsp black pepper

1/3 cup dried basil

1/3 cup dried oregano

1/2 cup olive oil

Directions:

Preheat oven to 300F. Combine all the spice in a bowl. Poke holes all over the roast. Stick some garlic into the holes. Heat the olive oil, in a large oven-proof dish.

Seal the meat on all sides and leave it aside in a plate. Coat it with the spice mix. Drizzle olive oil on top of the roast and pat the oil over the seasonings.

Arrange the roast beef in the middle of the baking dish. Crush the remaining garlic and add it to the dish together with the onions, bay leaves, carrots, celery, rosemary and tomato paste.

Bake on lowest rack approximately 2 hours, uncovered, until the internal temperature reaches 140 F (160 F for well done). Remove from oven and set aside, to cool for about 20 to 30 minutes.

Mediterranean Steak with Olives and Mushrooms

Serves 4

Ingredients:

1 lb boneless beef sirloin steak, 3/4-inch thick, cut into 4 pieces

1 large red onion, chopped

1 cup mushrooms

4 garlic cloves, thinly sliced

4 tablespoons olive oil

1/2 cup green olives, coarsely chopped

1 cup parsley leaves, finely cut

Directions:

Heat 2 tablespoons of olive oil in a large skillet over medium-high heat. Add the beef and cook until well browned on both sides. Remove the beef from the skillet and pour off excess fat.

Heat the remaining oil in the skillet. Add the onion and garlic and cook for 2-3 minutes, stirring occasionally.

Add the mushrooms and olives and cook until the mushrooms are done, stirring often.

Return the beef to the skillet. Reduce heat to medium. Cover and cook the beef for 3-4 minutes. Stir in parsley and serve.

Beef Stew with Quince

Serves 6-8

Ingredients:

2 lbs chuck roast, trimmed of fat and cut into 2 inch pieces

2 onions, chopped

2-3 tomatoes, pureed

1-2 bay leaves

1 cinnamon stick

3 quinces, peeled, cored and cubed

5-6 prunes

1 tsp paprika

1 tsp salt

1/2 tsp black pepper

1 tbsp raw honey

6 tbsp olive oil

Directions:

Heat half the olive oil in a large pot over medium-high heat. Seal the meat in batches, then set it aside in a plate. Sauté the onions for 6-8 minutes.

Add the meat back to the pot. Add the bay leaves, cinnamon, tomato puree, salt, pepper, and enough water to cover the meat. Stir and bring the pot to a simmer.

Heat remaining olive oil in a skillet and sauté the quince for 3-4 minutes until the edges start to caramelize. Add the quince to the stew pot along with the prunes and honey.

Stir, cover, and simmer for two hours over low heat. Stir occasionally and make sure there is enough liquid in the pot. If it looks dry, add some water.

Before serving discard the bay leaves and cinnamon stick.

Mediterranean Beef Casserole

Serves 6

Ingredients:

2 lbs lean steak, cut into large pieces

3 onions, sliced

4 garlic cloves, cut

2 red peppers, cut

1 green pepper, cut

1 zucchini, cut

3 tomatoes, quartered

2 tbsp tomato paste or purée

1/2 cup green olives, pitted

1/2 cup of water

1 tsp dry oregano

salt and black pepper, to taste

Directions:

Heat the olive oil in a deep baking dish and seal the beef. Add all vegetables and stir.

Dilute the tomato paste in half a cup of water and pour it over the meat mixture.

Season well and bake, covered, in a preheated to 350 F for one hour.

Beef and Onion Stew

Serves 6

Ingredients:

2 lbs lean beef, cubed

3 lbs shallots, peeled

5 garlic cloves, peeled, whole

3 tbsp tomato paste

1 bay leaves

1/4 cup of olive oil

3 tbsp lemon juice

1 tsp salt

Directions:

Heat a stew pot and brown the meat in olive oil. Add remaining ingredients and enough water to cover everything.

Bring to a boil. Reduce heat to low, cover, and simmer for 1-2 hours, stirring occasionally, until beef is cooked through.

Beef with Mushrooms

Serves 4

Ingredients:

1 lb stewing beef

2 cups mushrooms, sliced

2 leeks, chopped

4 garlic cloves, sliced

3 tbsp olive oil

2 tbsp tomato paste or purée

1/2 cup water

1/2 cup dry red wine

1 tsp paprika

1 tsp dried thyme

1 tsp salt

black pepper, to taste

Directions:

Heat the olive oil in a large pot and seal the beef pieces very well. Add in the leeks and the garlic and cook over low heat until the beef pieces are tender. Add sugar, paprika, thyme, salt and pepper and stir.

Dilute the tomato paste in half a cup of hot water. Pour it over the meat, stir and add the mushrooms. Cover and simmer, stirring from time to time, over medium-low heat for 40 minutes.

Uncover and simmer some more until the liquid has evaporated.

Beef and Spinach Stew

Serves 4

Ingredients:

1 lb stewing beef

10 oz frozen spinach

1 onion, chopped

3 garlic cloves, crushed

1 cup beef broth

1/2 cup canned tomatoes, drained

4 tbsp olive oil

1 tbsp paprika

salt and pepper, to taste

Directions:

In a large stew pot, heat the olive oil and seal the beef pieces. Add onion and garlic and sauté for a few minutes.

Add paprika, beef broth and bring to the boil then reduce heat and simmer, covered, for 30-40 minutes. Add the tomatoes and spinach.

Stir and cook, uncovered, for 10 minutes.

Cabbage and Beef Stew

Serves 6-8

Ingredients:

1 lb stewing beef

1 medium cabbage, cut into thin strips

1 onion, chopped

1 carrot, chopped

1 red bell pepper, cut into strips

2 tomatoes, chopped

1 tsp paprika

1/2 tsp cumin

1/2 tsp cinnamon

4 tbsp olive oil

1 1/2 cups water

Directions:

Heat a large pot over medium-high heat and brown the cubed beef in 2 tbsp of olive oil. Add 1 1/2 cups of water and bring to the boil then reduce heat and simmer for an hour or until the meat is almost done.

In another pot heat the remaining olive oil and sauté the onions and carrot until soft. Add the red pepper and stir, add the cabbage, tomatoes and spice and stir some more.

Combine the meat and the cabbage mixture and bring to the boil. Reduce heat and simmer for 30 minutes or until the cabbage is cooked through.

Beef and Okra Stew

Serves 6-8

Ingredients:

1 lb stew meat

1 lb frozen okra

1 onion, chopped

3 garlic cloves, crushed

1 cup canned tomatoes, diced

3 tbsp tomato purée

1/2 tsp cumin

1/2 tsp dried coriander

1 cup water

4 tbsp olive oil

salt and pepper to taste

Directions:

In a large saucepan, heat olive oil and seal meat. Add onions and garlic and sauté, stirring, for 2-3 minutes. Add tomatoes, cumin, coriander, salt and pepper. Add water and tomato purée. Stir and combine well.

Add okra and bring to a boil, then reduce heat to low and simmer, covered, for an hour or until meat is tender and done.

Uncover and simmer for five more minutes.

Mixed Vegetables with Beef

Serves 6-8

Ingredients:

2 lb stew beef

2 eggplants, cubed

1 zucchini, cubed

2 red peppers, cut

1 onion, sliced

4 garlic cloves, cut

3 tomatoes, diced

1 cup parsley leaves, chopped

1/4 cup olive oil

1 tsp paprika

salt, to taste

black pepper, to taste

Directions:

Sprinkle the eggplant pieces with salt and set aside in a strainer for 15 minutes. Wash the salt and the excess juices and pat dry the eggplant pieces.

Heat the olive oil in a large pot and sauté the beef pieces for a few minutes until well browned. Add in the vegetables, stirring. Add paprika, salt and pepper and stir very well again.

Transfer the meat and vegetables to an oven proof dish and bake in a preheated to 305 F oven for an hour.

Sprinkle with parsley and serve.

Paleo Stuffed Peppers

Serves 6

Ingredients:

8 red or green bell peppers, cored and seeded

2 lbs ground beef

1 onion, finely cut

2 tomatoes, grated

a bunch of fresh parsley, chopped

3 tbsp olive oil

1 tbsp paprika

Directions:

Heat the oil and sauté the onion for 2-3 minutes. Remove from heat. Add paprika, ground beef, tomatoes, and season with salt and pepper.

Combine very well and stuff each pepper with the mixture using a spoon. Every pepper should be 3/4 full.

Arrange the peppers in a deep oven proof dish and top up with warm water to half fill the dish.

Cover and bake for about 40-50 minutes at 350 F.

Stuffed Artichokes

Serves 6

Ingredients:

1 lb lean ground beef

6 large firm fresh artichokes

1 onion, grated

2 garlic cloves, chopped

4 tomatoes, grated

5 tbsp olive oil

1/2 cup parsley leaves, very finely cut

1 tsp paprika

salt and pepper, to taste

juice of 1/2 lemon

Directions:

Peel artichokes and cut off tips. With the help of a spoon, carve out the center of artichokes. Put artichokes in a large bowl together with a teaspoon of salt, lemon juice and enough water to cover them completely.

Heat olive oil in a cooking pot and sauté onions and garlic until transparent. Add in ground beef, parsley and paprika. Cook for 5 minutes, stirring. Add tomatoes and cook until almost all liquid evaporates. Season with salt and pepper and remove from heat.

Wash and drain artichokes. Stuff artichokes with the already cooled mixture and arrange them in a cooking pot in one layer.

Add 2 cups water and bring to the boil then reduce heat and simmer for about 40 minutes.

Ground Beef Stuffed Cabbage Leaves

Serves 8

Ingredients:

1 lb ground beef

20 medium sized pickled cabbage leaves

1 onion, diced

1 leek, finely cut

2 tsp tomato paste

2 tsp paprika

1 tsp dried mint

½ tsp black pepper

1/3 cup olive oil

salt to taste

Directions:

Sauté the onion and leek in the oil for about 2-3 minutes. Remove from heat and add the beef, tomato paste, paprika, mint, black pepper. Add salt only if the cabbage leaves are not too salty. Mix everything very well.

In a large pot place a few cabbage leaves on the base. Place a cabbage leaf on a large plate with the thickest part closest to you. Spoon 1-2 teaspoons of the meat mixture and fold over each edge to create a tight sausage-like parcel. Place in the pot in two or three layers.

Cover with a few cabbage leaves and pour over some boiling water so that the water level remains lower than the top layer of cabbage leaves. Top with a small dish upside down to prevent scattering. Bring to the boil, then lower the heat and cook for around an hour.

Meatballs in Tomato Sauce

Serves 6

Ingredients:

2 lbs ground beef

2 onions, grated

1 carrot, chopped

2 garlic cloves, cut

3-4 white mushrooms, sliced

1/3 cup parsley leaves, finely chopped, for the meatballs

3 cups canned tomatoes, diced

1/2 cup chicken broth

1/2 cup parsley leaves, to serve

Directions:

Combine ground beef, finely cut onion, parsley, salt and pepper in a large bowl. Roll tablespoonfuls of mince mixture into balls.

Place meatballs on a tray lined with baking paper. Cover and set aside.

Heat oil in a deep frying pan. Sauté finely cut onion, carrot and garlic for 2- 3 minutes, stirring. Add mushrooms and stir again.

Add tomatoes and broth and bring slowly to the boil over medium heat. Drop meatballs into tomato mixture.

Reduce heat to low and simmer, uncovered, for 30 minutes or until meatballs are cooked through.

Sprinkle with parsley, set aside for 5 minutes, and serve.

Small Beef Meatballs

Serves 6

Ingredients:

1 lb ground beef

1 onion, grated

1 egg, lightly whisked

1/4 cup parsley leaves, finely cut

2 garlic cloves, crushed

1 tsp dried mint

2 tsp dried oregano

1/4 cup olive oil

Directions:

Combine meat, onion, egg, parsley, mint, garlic and oregano. Mix very well with hands. Roll tablespoonfuls of the meat mixture into balls.

Heat oil in a frying pan over medium-high heat. Cook meatballs in batches, turning, for 6-7 minutes or until cooked through.

Transfer to a serving plate. Serve with vegetable salad or stewed vegetables.

Meatloaf with Vegetables

Serves 6-8

Ingredients:

2 lbs ground beef

2 eggs, lightly beaten

5-6 zucchinis, diced

1 eggplant, peeled and diced

5-6 tomatoes, diced

1 cup chicken broth

3 tbsp olive oil

1/2 cup fresh parsley, finely cut

1 tsp black pepper

1/2 tsp salt

Directions:

Combine ground beef, eggs, olive oil, parsley, salt, and pepper in a bowl and mix with hands. Make a loaf and arrange it in the center of a baking dish.

Peel and cut eggplant and zucchinis. Puree tomatoes. Arrange vegetables around the meatloaf, season with salt, add 1 cup of chicken broth and stir. Bake in a preheated to 350 F oven for 1 hour. If necessary cover the meat with foil.

Beef Kebabs

Serves 4

Ingredients:

2 lbs ground beef

2 onions, grated

1 tsp cumin

1 tsp dried oregano

1 tsp dried parsley

Directions:

Preheat a barbecue or char grill on medium-high. Combine the ground beef, onions and herbs in a bowl.

Roll tablespoonfuls of the mixture into balls. Thread 4-5 meatballs onto 1 skewer. Repeat to make 12 kebabs.

Cook the kebabs for about 2-3 minutes each side for medium cooked. Transfer to a plate, cover with foil and set aside for 5 minutes to rest.

Pork Roast and Cabbage

Serves 4

Ingredients:

2 cups of cooked pork roast, chopped

1/2 head of cabbage

2 onions, chopped

1 lemon, juice only

1 tomato, chopped

1 tsp paprika

1/2 tsp cumin

black pepper, to taste

2 tbsp olive oil

Directions:

Heat olive oil and sauté cabbage, pork and onions. Add cumin, paprika, lemon juice, tomato and stir.

Cover and cook until vegetables are tender.

Orange Pork Chops

Serves 4

Ingredients:

4 pork chops, about 4 oz each

1 onion, thinly sliced

4 garlic cloves, crushed

1/4 tsp cumin

1/4 tsp oregano

1 tsp black pepper

1 tbsp raw honey

1/2 cup orange juice

5 tbsp olive oil

Directions:

Crush the garlic, oregano, black pepper and cumin together into a paste. Rub each chop with the garlic paste then place in a glass bowl.

Dilute one tbsp of honey into the orange juice and pour it over the chops. Add the onions, stir and cover. Set aside to marinate for at least one hour.

Remove the chops from the marinade and pat dry. Heat oil over medium high heat and brown the chops on both sides. Arrange them in a baking dish and add marinade and onions.

Bake in a preheated to 350 F on for 20 minutes or until the chops are cooked through.

Pork Skewers

Serves 6

Ingredients:

6 (2 lbs) pork loin medallions, cut into 2 inch cubes

2 red or green peppers, deseeded, cut into 2 inch pieces

30 white mushrooms, whole

Directions:

Preheat barbecue or char grill on medium-high. Thread pork, peppers and mushrooms onto 1 skewer. Repeat to make 12 skewers.

Cook them for about 2-3 minutes each side for medium cooked. Transfer to a plate, cover with foil and set aside for 5 minutes to rest.

Broccoli Bacon Frittata

Serves 4

Ingredients:

4 eggs

2 tbsp canned coconut milk

1 cup broccoli florets

3 spring onions, finely chopped

3 strips bacon, cooked and crumbled

1 large tomato, sliced

2 tbsp olive oil

salt and black pepper to taste

Directions:

Steam broccoli florets until soft. Beat eggs, coconut milk, salt and pepper.

Heat olive oil in a medium baking dish. Add broccoli and bacon and stir. Cook for 1 minute. Pour over egg mixture and stir again. Add in spring onions.

Cover with sliced tomato and bake in a preheated to 350 F oven for 15 minutes.

Roasted Brussels Sprouts with Bacon and Onions

Serves 6

Ingredients:

4 strips bacon

2 tbsp olive oil

1 lb Brussels sprouts, halved

1 large onion, chopped

salt and freshly ground black pepper, to taste

Directions:

Cook bacon in a large skillet over medium-high heat until crispy. Transfer to a plate, then chop.

In the same pan, add onions and Brussels Sprouts and cook, stirring occasionally, until sprouts are golden brown.

Season with salt and pepper to taste and toss bacon back into pan.

Roast Lamb Leg with Herbs

Serves 4

Ingredients:

1 leg of lamb

3 garlic cloves, crushed

1 tsp black pepper

1 bay leaf

1 tsp mint

1/2 tsp thyme

1/2 tsp sage

2 tbsp olive oil

Directions:

Mix garlic, seasonings, herbs and oil together. Rub on the lamb leg.

Place on rack in roasting pan. Cook, uncovered, at 300F for approximately two hours or until cooked through.

Lamb-Asparagus Stew

Serves 6

Ingredients:

1 lb lamb meat, cubed

2 lbs fresh asparagus, trimmed and cut into 2 inch pieces

1 onion, chopped

3 tbsp olive oil

1 cup water

juice of 1 lemon

1 tsp dry mint

1 tsp dry oregano

Wash and trim asparagus. Cut into 2 inch pieces.

Directions:

Heat olive oil in a deep skillet. Sauté lamb pieces until browned. Add onions and cook some more. Add water, spices, cover and cook for an hour or until tender.

Add asparagus and cook for 15 more minutes. Add lemon juice and serve.

Spring Lamb Stew

Serves 6

Ingredients:

11/2 lb lamb meat, cubed

1 lb mushrooms, chopped

1 onion, cut

2 bunches fresh spring onions, cut

2 tomatoes, chopped

3 tbsp olive oil

1 tsp paprika

a bunch of fresh mint, finely cut

2 bunches of fresh parsley, finely cut

Directions:

Heat olive oil in a deep skillet. Sauté lamb pieces until browned. Add onions and cook some more. Add paprika, cover and cook for an hour or until tender.

Add spring onions, mushrooms, tomatoes, mint and parsley and simmer for 10-15 more minutes.

Uncover and cook for a few more minutes, until the liquid evaporates.

Salmon Kebabs

Serves 4

Ingredients:

2 shallots, ends trimmed, halved

6 skinless salmon fillets, cut into 1 inch pieces

3 limes, cut into thin wedges

Directions:

Preheat barbecue or char grill on medium-high. Thread shallot, salmon and lime wedges onto each skewer. Repeat to make 12 kebabs.

Bake the kebabs for about 3 minutes each side for medium cooked. Transfer to a plate, cover with foil and set aside for 5 minutes to rest.

Serve with vegetable salad or stewed vegetables.

Swordfish Kebabs

Serves 4

Ingredients:

2 zucchinis, cut in 2 inch cubes

2 lbs skinless swordfish steaks, cut into 2 inch cubes

1 cup cherry tomatoes

1/2 cup basil leaves, finely chopped

4 garlic cloves, crushed

1 lemon, juiced

rind from 1 lemon

olive oil cooking spray

Directions:

Prepare marinade by combining garlic, lemon rind, lemon juice, basil leaves, salt and pepper in a small bowl.

Thread fish cubes onto skewers, then zucchinis and tomatoes. Place skewers in a shallow plate. Brush with marinade and refrigerate for 30 minutes if time permits.

Spray skewers with olive oil spray and bake on a preheated barbecue plate on medium heat.

Bake for 6-7 minutes, turning, or until fish is just cooked through.

Roasted Butternut Squash

Serves 4

Ingredients:

1/2 butternut squash, peeled, seeds removed, flesh chopped

2 sprigs fresh rosemary

2 garlic cloves, finely chopped

2 tbsp olive oil

salt and freshly ground black pepper, to taste

Directions:

Preheat the oven to 350 F. Place the butternut squash pieces on a baking tray and scatter over the rosemary and the chopped garlic.

Drizzle with the olive oil and season, to taste, with salt and freshly ground black pepper.

Transfer to the oven and roast for 12-15 minutes, or until the squash is tender and golden-brown.

Roasted Artichoke Hearts

Serves 4

Ingredients:

2 cans artichoke hearts

4 garlic cloves, quartered

2 tsp olive oil

1 tsp dried savory

salt and pepper, to taste

2-3 tbsp lemon juice, to serve

Directions:

Preheat oven to 375°F. Drain artichoke hearts, rinse them well and place them in a bowl. Toss in garlic, savory and olive oil.

Place artichoke hearts in a baking dish and bake for about 45 minutes tossing a few times if desired.

Season with salt and pepper, and serve with lemon juice.

Beet Fries

Serves 4

Ingredients:

3 red beets, cut

1 tbsp olive oil

a bunch of spring onions, finely cut

2 cloves of garlic, crushed

1 tsp salt

Directions:

Line a baking dish with baking paper. Wash and peel the beets then cut them in strips similar to French fries.

Toss the beets with the olive oil, spring onions, garlic and salt and arrange them on a the baking sheet.

Bake in a preheated to 425 F oven for 25-30 minutes, flipping halfway through.

Grilled Vegetable Skewers

Serves 4

Ingredients:

1 red pepper

1 green pepper

4 slim zucchinis, sliced

3 onions, quartered

12 medium mushrooms, whole

2 garlic cloves, crushed

1 spring fresh rosemary

salt and ground black pepper

2 tbsp olive oil

Directions:

Deseed and cut the peppers into chunks. Divide between 6 skewers threading alternately with the zucchinis, onions and mushrooms.

Set aside the skewers in a shallow plate.

Mix the crushed garlic and the herbs, salt, pepper and the olive oil. Roll each skewer in the mixture.

Bake them on a hot barbecue or char grill, turning occasionally, until slightly charred.

Paleo Breakfast Recipes

Mediterranean Omelette with Fennel, Olives, and Dill

Serves 6

Ingredients:

2 cups fresh fennel bulb, sliced and chopped

1 cup cherry tomatoes, halved

1/4 cup green olives, pitted

5 eggs, gently beaten with salt, black pepper and paprika

2 tbsp olive oil

1/2 tsp ground black pepper

1 tsp paprika

1/2 tsp salt

2 tbsp chopped fresh dill

Directions:

Heat one tablespoon of olive oil in a nonstick pan over medium-high heat. Sauté the fennel bulb, stirring, for 3-4 minutes, or until light brown.

Cover and simmer until soft, about 5 minutes. Add tomatoes and olives. Season with salt and pepper. Transfer fennel mixture to a bowl.

Heat the remaining oil in the same skillet and cook eggs until just set in center, tilting the skillet and lifting edges with a spatula in a way to let uncooked portion flow underneath.

Cover with fennel mixture and sprinkle with dill. With the help of a spatula, fold uncovered half of omelette over; slide onto plate.

Spinach Omelette

Serves 4

Ingredients:

1 cup fresh spinach, chopped

5 spring onions, chopped

1/2 cup mushrooms, chopped

3 eggs, gently beaten

1/2 tsp salt

black pepper, to taste

Directions:

Heat olive oil in a large skillet. Gently sauté chopped vegetables.

Beat eggs with salt and black pepper in a bowl.

Pour them over the vegetables and cook until firm. Flip omelette and cook the other side.

Artichoke Frittata

Serves 4

Ingredients:

4 eggs

3 egg whites

1 tbsp canned coconut milk

1 tbsp olive oil

1 can artichoke hearts, chopped and drained

Directions:

Heat olive oil in a large non-stick pan and sauté artichokes. Beat eggs and egg whites together with a spoon of coconut milk and pour them over artichokes.

Bake in a preheated to 350 F oven until golden on top.

Avocado and Pumpkin Muffins

Serves 12

Ingredients:

1/2 cup mashed avocado

1 cup unsweetened pumpkin puree

3 large eggs

21/2 cups almond flour or almond meal

3 tbsp agave nectar or maple syrup

¾ tsp baking soda

1 tsp vinegar

½ tsp fine sea salt

1 tsp citrus zest

1 tsp cinnamon

1 tsp vanilla

2 tbsp vegetable oil

1 cup blueberries or diced apple

Directions:

Preheat oven to 375 F. Grease 12 muffin tin wells or line with paper cups.

In a large bowl, whisk the eggs, pumpkin, agave nectar, avocado, oil and vinegar. Add all extracts and citrus zest.

In a separate bowl, whisk the almond flour, baking soda and salt. Combine with avocado mixture; do not over-mix. Stir in blueberries.

Spoon batter into prepared muffin tin and bake for 14-18 minutes until set at the centers and golden brown at the edges.

Move the tin to a cooling rack and let muffins cool in the tin 30 minutes then serve.

The Perfect Coconut Flour Pancakes

Serves 8-9

Ingredients:

1/4 cup coconut flour

1/8 tsp baking soda

a pinch of salt

1/3 cup coconut milk

2 tbsp cold-pressed coconut oil

3 eggs

1-2 tbsp honey

1 tsp lemon zest

1 tsp vanilla extract

Maple syrup, to serve

butter for cooking

Directions:

In a bowl, mix the eggs, coconut oil, and honey together. Add in the coconut milk, vanilla extract, coconut flour, baking soda, lemon zest, and salt.

Combine everything well but don't over mix it. Melt a dab of butter in a skillet and using a measuring cup, add a little batter to the pan.

Check the underside of the pancake before flipping. Serve pancakes right away with maple syrup.

About the Author

Vesela lives in Bulgaria with her family of six (including the Jack Russell Terrier). Her passion is going green in everyday life and she loves to prepare homemade cosmetic and beauty products for all her family and friends.

Vesela has been publishing her cookbooks for over a year now. If you want to see other healthy family recipes that she has published, together with some natural beauty books, you can check out her <u>Author Page</u> on Amazon.

82705070R00076

Made in the USA
Lexington, KY
05 March 2018